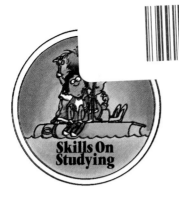

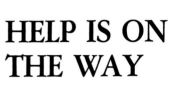

Skills On Studying

HELP IS ON THE WAY FOR:

Taking Notes

Written by Marilyn Berry
Pictures by Bartholomew

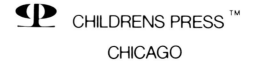

CHILDRENS PRESS ™

CHICAGO

Childrens Press
School and Library Edition

Executive Producer: Joy Berry
Editors: Nancy Cochran, Susan Motycka and Kate Dickey
Consultants: Kathleen McBride, Maureen Dryden and Donna Fisher
Design: Abigail Johnston
Typesetting: Curt Chelin

ISBN 0-516-03239-9
Copyright © 1985 by Marilyn Berry
Living Skills Press, Sebastopol, CA
Printed in the United States of America

So you need to start **taking notes.**

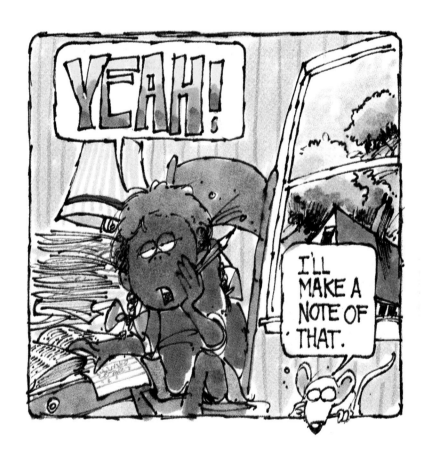

Hang on! Help is on the way!

If you have a hard time knowing how to take notes

- from a textbook,
- in class, and
- for special projects...

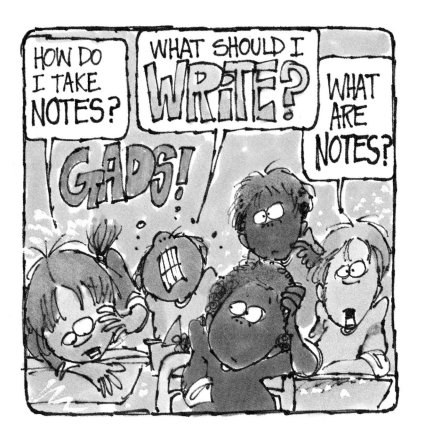

...you are not alone!

Just in case you're wondering...

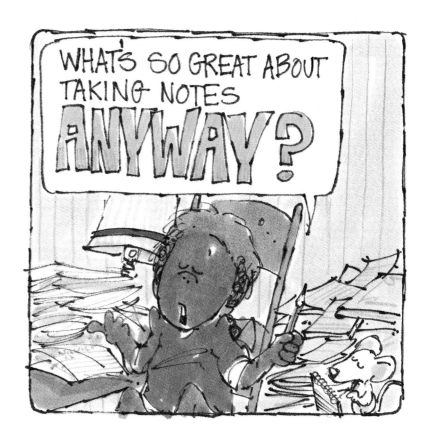

...why don't we start at the beginning?

What Is Notetaking?

A **note** is a brief record of acts or ideas.
When you take notes, you are writing down
important information.

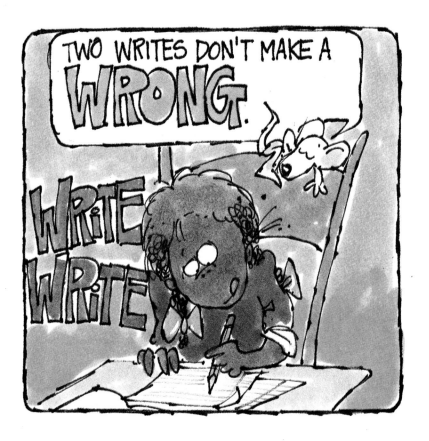

A note is also a reminder of information you have read or heard. You are expected to remember a large amount of information every day. If you learn to take notes, you will be able to recall a lot more of that information.

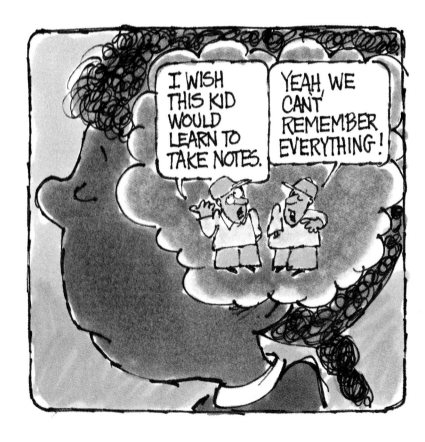

Why Is Taking Notes Important?

Learning to take notes can help you in everyday life. Here are two examples:

- Taking notes helps you remember important dates.

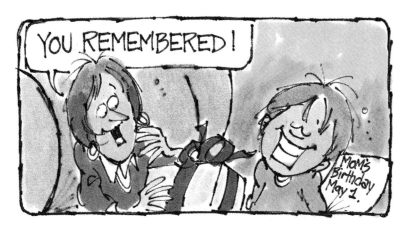

- Taking notes helps you remember thoughts and ideas.

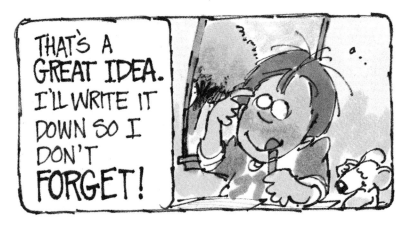

Learning to take notes can help you in school. Here are two examples:

• Taking notes helps you study for tests.

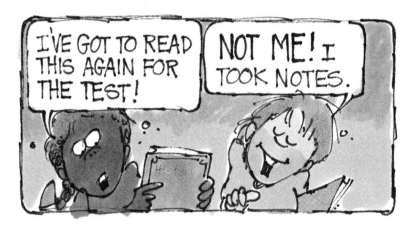

• Taking notes helps you gather information for school projects.

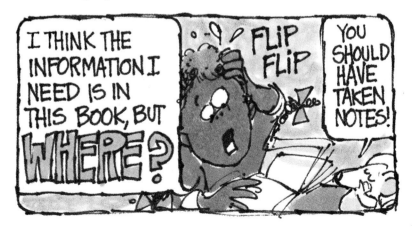

The older you get and the more you go to school, the more you will find that taking notes is an important skill. Notetaking becomes easier with practice. But first you need to learn about the best methods for taking notes.

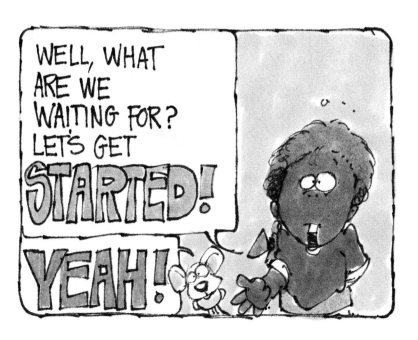

Writing Notes to Yourself

There are many important details that you need to remember during a school day. You do not need to memorize them all. Learn to write notes to yourself as a reminder. Here are some examples:

Lists of "Things to Do"
Keep a page in your notebook of "Things to Do." When there is a task that you need to do, write it down on your list. As you complete each task, cross it off your list.

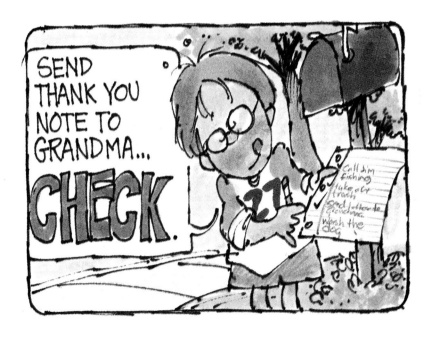

Assignment Book

Keep a special notebook, just for assignments. As each assignment in class is given, write it in this notebook. Be sure to include this information:

- the subject
- the due date
- books and materials needed
- details of the assignment
- a sample problem, if possible

Keeping an assignment book will help you remember your homework.

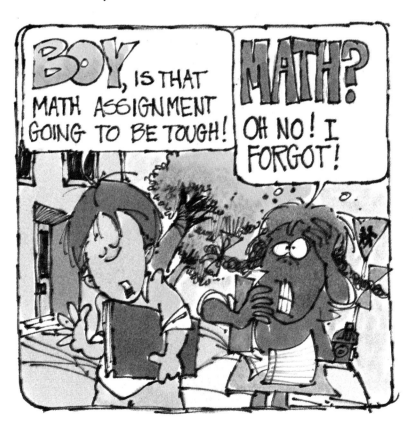

Idea File

When you think of a creative idea, write it down so you don't forget it. You might not need the idea at that moment, but it could come in handy later. Keep a file of ideas for such assignments as

- written reports,
- creative writing,
- special projects, and
- art work.

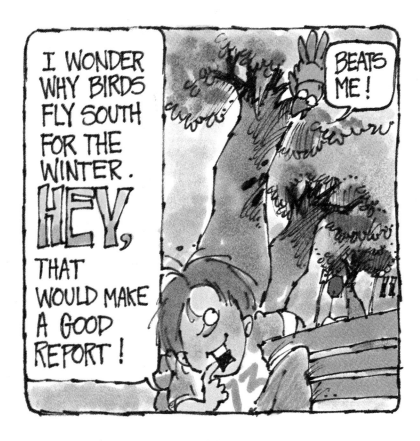

Taking Notes for School

The hardest part of taking notes is deciding what to write down. The key is to pick out the most important facts and ideas and to leave out the information that is not important. But sometimes it is hard to decide what is important and what is not.

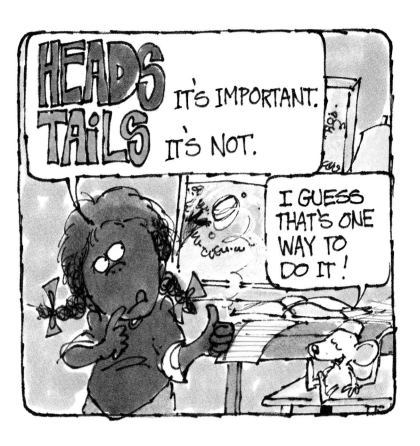

There are two basic rules that can help you decide if a piece of information is important or not. Remember these rules as you take notes.

RULE ONE

The information is important and should be included in your notes if it
- helps you answer a question about the topic you are studying, or
- helps you understand the topic more clearly.

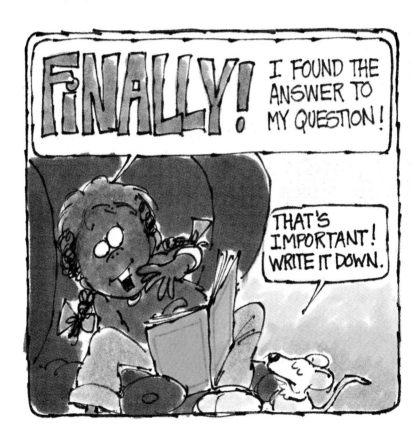

RULE TWO.

The information is *not* important and does not
need to be included in your notes if it
- repeats something that has already been said
  about the topic you are studying, or
- does not help you understand the topic more
  clearly.

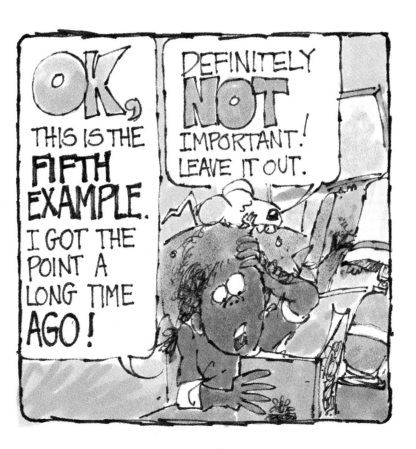

USING YOUR OWN STYLE

Everyone develops his or her own style of taking notes. As you continue to take notes, you will develop your own style, too. Here are some ideas:
- Use either whole sentences or short phrases.
- Learn how to shorten words that are used often. For example, use "trans" for transportation.
- Use initials for names that are used often.
- Learn to be brief but not so brief you can't understand your own notes.

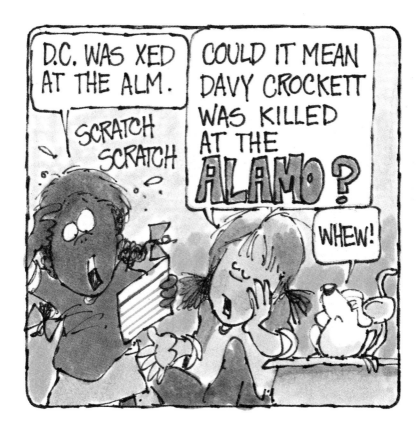

DAILY SCHOOLWORK

There will be times as you do your daily school-work when taking notes will be very helpful. Taking notes helps you

- keep track of the information you are expected to learn,
- pick out the information you don't understand so you can ask questions,
- be prepared for class, and
- study for tests.

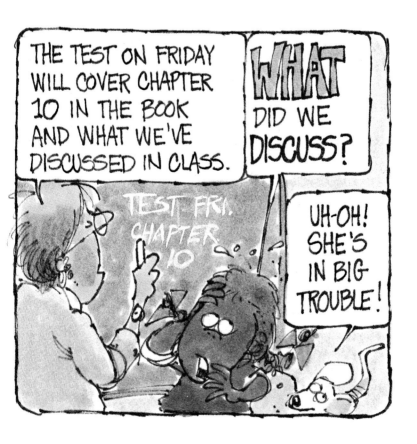

Keeping a Notebook

It's a lot easier to take notes and keep track of them if you use a notebook. You can have a separate notebook for each of your school subjects. Or, you might want to keep all your notes in one binder with a section for each subject. No matter which of these methods you choose, it is important that you

- have a notebook available for taking notes, and
- know where to find your notes when you need them.

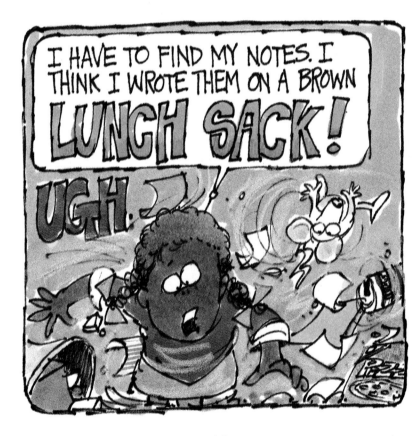

Taking Notes from a Textbook

When your teacher gives you a reading assignment in a textbook, you will learn more if you take notes as you read. Try following these five simple steps.

Step one: Look over the assignment.
- Read the title and the introduction.
- Read any phrases or words in bold type.
- Look at the illustrations and their captions.
- Read the conclusion.

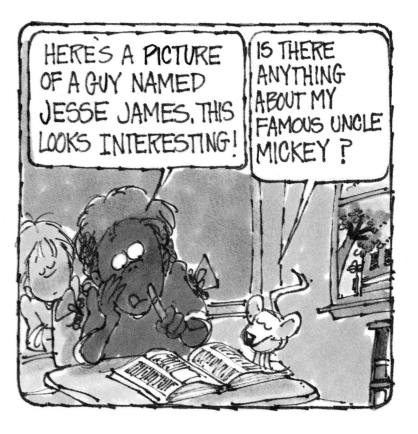

Step two: Ask questions.

- Look at the questions at the end of each chapter. They will tell you what important information to look for as you read.
- Or, write down several of your own questions that came to mind as you looked over the assignment.

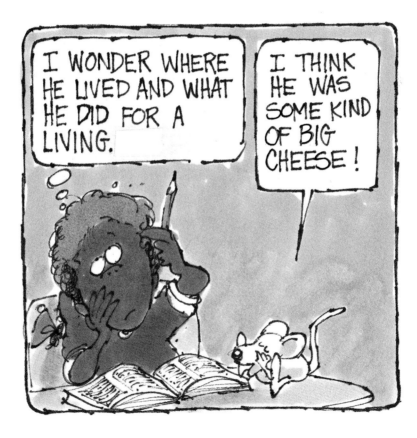

Step three: Read the assignment.
- As you read, think about your questions.
- When you come to some information that answers a question or seems important, carefully mark the place with a paper clip. (Remember the two rules of notetaking.)

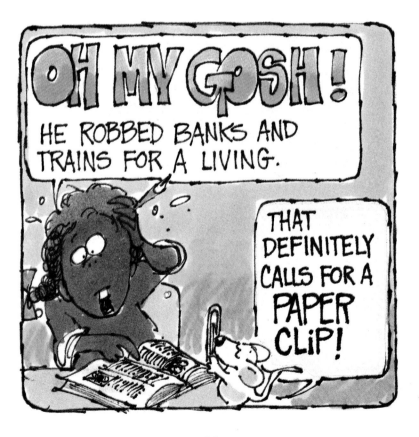

Step four: Answer the questions.
- After you have read the assignment, close your book and try to answer all of the questions.
- Write down the answers in the proper section of your notebook.

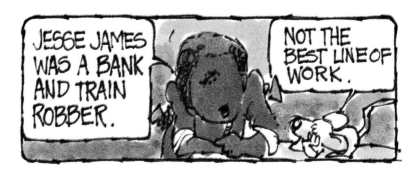

Step five: Check your answers.
- Check your answers to make sure they are right and correct any mistakes.
- Check each place you marked to make sure you wrote down all the important information.
  Be sure to remove all your markers.
- Save your notes and study them for future tests.

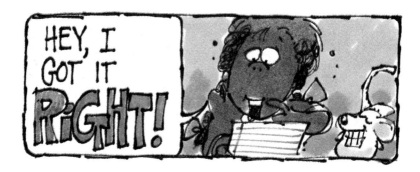

Taking Notes in Class

Throughout the day, your teacher explains a lot of important information to your class. It would help you remember this information if you wrote down some notes. Taking notes in class is easy if you are prepared and know how to do it.

Be Prepared
- Always have your notebook and a sharpened pencil ready.
- Make sure you can hear the teacher clearly.
- Make sure you can see the chalkboard.

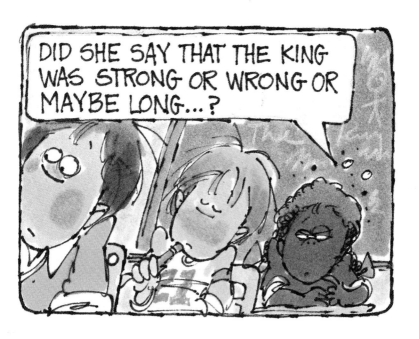

How to Take Notes in Class
1. Turn to the proper section in your notebook. Write the date and the topic at the top of a clean page.
2. Listen and watch for clues of important points such as:
   - "Today we're going to discuss..."
   - "This is important..."
   - "Please remember this..."
   - A point that is repeated several times
   - Anything written on the chalkboard
3. Write down only important facts and ideas.
4. Ask questions when you do not understand something.

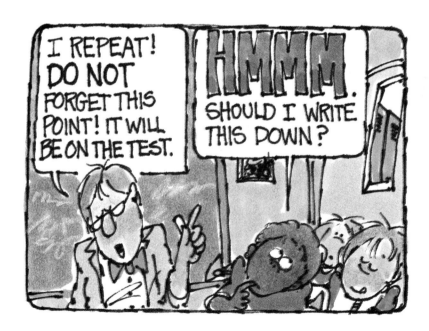

Copy Your Notes

Many times when you take notes in class, you need to write down the information quickly. Your notes might be messy and disorganized. If so, copy your notes onto a clean piece of paper at the end of the day. This will help you

- review the information that was discussed,
- sort out any information you don't understand (be sure to have your teacher explain these items), and
- organize your notes for future studying.

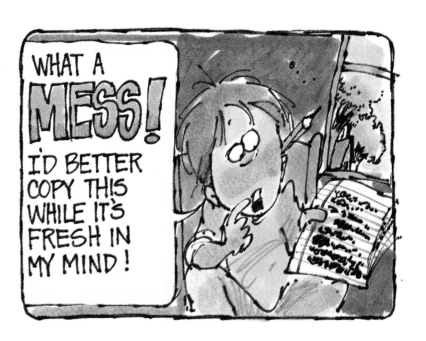

SPECIAL RESEARCH PROJECTS

There will be times in school when your teacher will assign special projects that require some research. For these projects, you will be gathering a lot of information from several different resources. To help you keep it all straight, you will need to study a system of notetaking and follow it carefully.

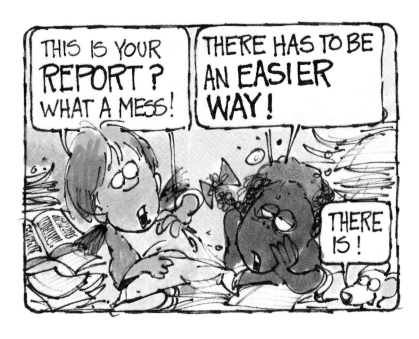

There are three notetaking systems which you can use when gathering information for a project. You can use
- note cards,
- topic sheets, or
- a note chart.

Each system works in a different way. You might want to try each one once to see which system works best for you.

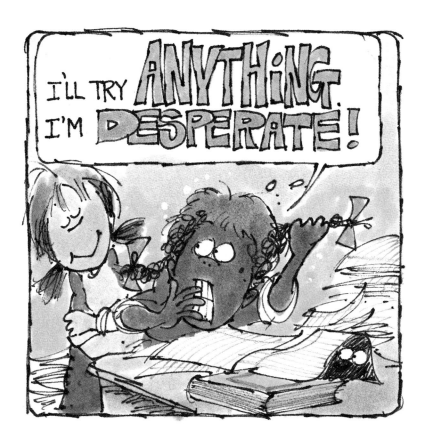

Note Cards

The use of note cards is a popular system of notetaking. As you do your research, you simply write down any information you need on 3'' x 5'' or 4'' x 6'' index cards. Once you have gathered all the information for your project, the cards can then be easily arranged and rearranged into any order you choose.

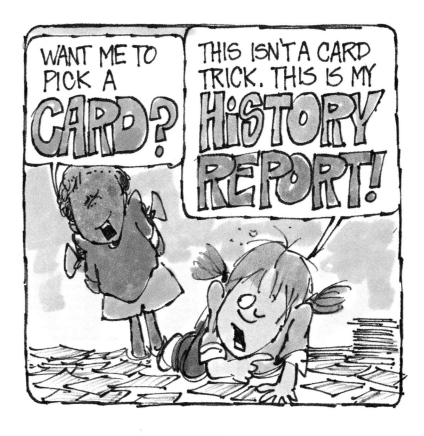

When using note cards for your research, there are some important rules to follow:

- Write only on one side of the card.
- Identify your resource on every card (such as the title and author of a book).
- Write down the location of the information (such as a page number).
- Put only one complete fact, idea, or quote on each card. Try to limit the information to one or two sentences.
- Number the main points of your project. Then assign the information on each card to one of your main points. Write the number of the main point at the top of the note card.

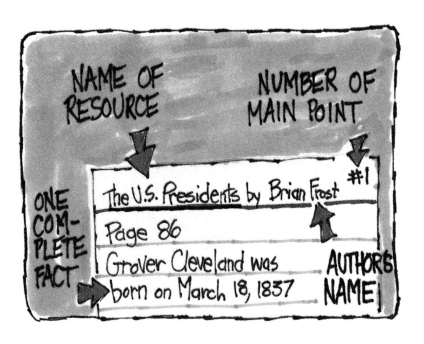

Bibliography Cards

As you gather information for your project,
it is important that you keep track of the
resources you use. Each resource should be
recorded on a separate card called a bibliography
card. This information will come in handy when
you need to

- look up information a second time,
- check a quotation, or
- prepare a bibliography (a list of the resources
  you used for your project).

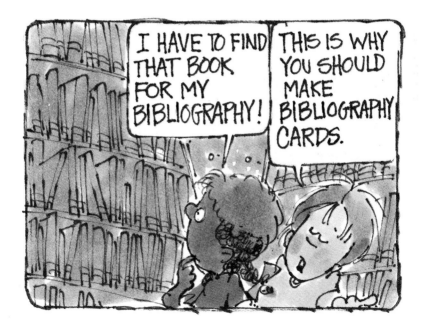

The information that you record on a bibliography card should include the same information you will need for your actual bibliography. If you use the proper form on your note cards, you will be able to copy the information right onto the bibliography page of your project. Here are the proper forms to use for three types of resources:

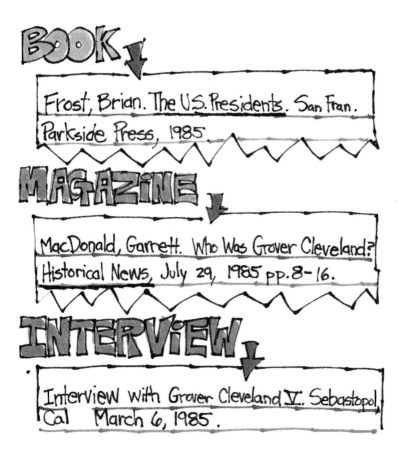

BOOK

Frost, Brian. The U.S. Presidents. San Fran. Parkside Press, 1985.

MAGAZINE

MacDonald, Garrett. Who Was Grover Cleveland? Historical News, July 29, 1985 pp. 8-16.

INTERVIEW

Interview with Grover Cleveland V. Sebastopol, Cal. March 6, 1985.

Topic Sheets

Using topic sheets is another good system of notetaking. Instead of using index cards, you write down any information you want to use on labeled sheets of paper. Each sheet of paper is labeled with one of the major points or topics of your project. All topic sheets are kept in a special notebook.

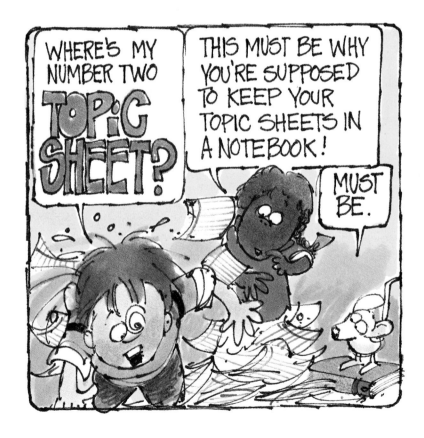

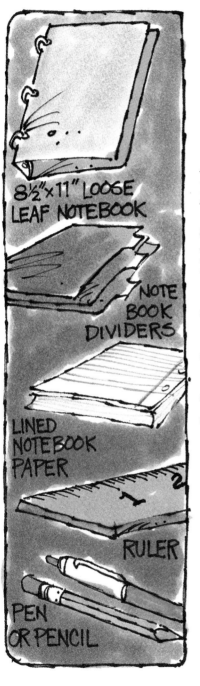

8½"×11" LOOSE LEAF NOTEBOOK

NOTE BOOK DIVIDERS

LINED NOTEBOOK PAPER

RULER

PEN OR PENCIL

Making Your Topic Sheets
To set up the topic sheet system for your project you will need

- an 8½'' x 11'' loose-leaf notebook,
- notebook dividers (one for each topic),
- several pages of lined notebook paper,
- a ruler, and
- a pen or pencil.

Instructions:

- Decide on the main points of your project and put them in a logical order.
- Write one main point on each of the notebook dividers and put them in the notebook.
- Draw a two-inch margin on the left side of three pieces of notebook paper.
- Write "Resources" above the left margin on each page.
- Write the title of the first point at the topic of each page and put them in your notebook.
- Make up topic sheets for each section of your notebook.

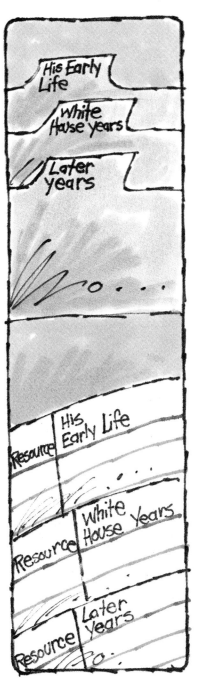

35

Using Your Topic Sheets

As you research your project, keep your notebook handy. When you find some information you can use, record it in your notebook.

- Determine which main point the information falls under.
- Turn to a topic sheet in that section of the notebook.
- In the left hand margin, identify the resource (such as the title, author and page number of a book).
- Write down the information you need on the topic sheet.
- Leave a space between notes.
- Use only one side of the page.

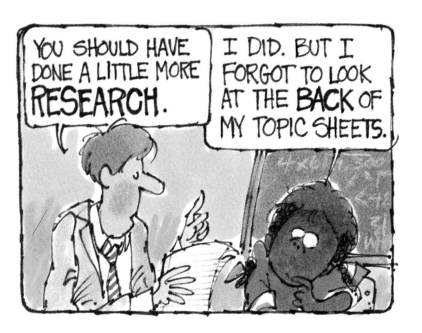

Bibliography Sheets

You will need to keep track of your resources, just as you would for the note card system. Write "Bibliography" on a separate sheet of paper and keep it in the back of your notebook. As you use a resource, record all the information you will need for the actual bibliography page of your project. Remember to use proper form.

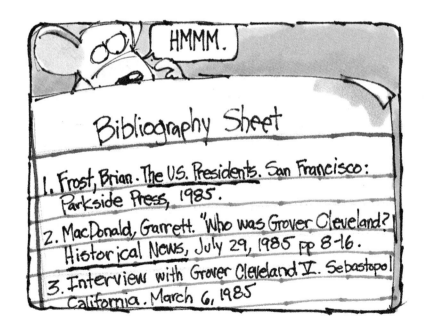

Note Chart

A note chart is not as portable as note cards or
topic sheets. However, a note chart displays your
whole project at once. This allows you to get an
overview of the project as it progresses.

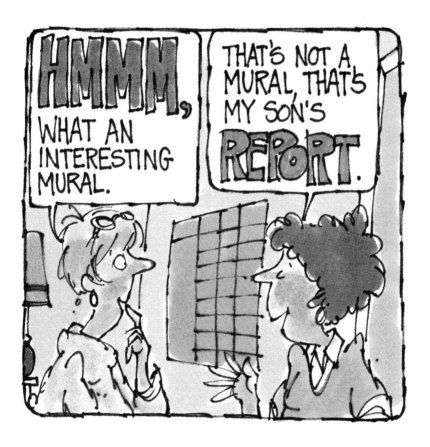

Making Your Note Chart

To set up the note chart system for your project you will need

- a piece of poster board (or a large piece of paper approximately 22'' x 28'',
- a yardstick, and
- a black marking pen.

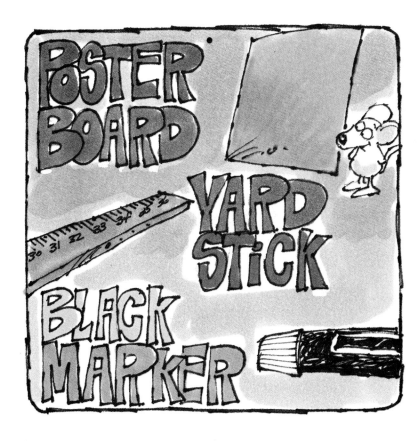

Instructions:

- Decide on the main points of your project and put them in a logical order.
- Using the yardstick and marking pen, divide the poster board into columns. There should be one column for resources and one for each main point of your report.
- At the top of the left hand column, write ''resources.''
- At the top of each remaining column, write one of the main points of your project.
- In each of the ''main point'' columns, make boxes large enough to write at least one or two sentences.

Resources	Early Years	White House Years	Later Years

A REAL WORK OF ART.

Using Your Note Chart

As you research your project, fill in your note chart with the information you want to use.

- When you use a resource, list it in the resource column of your chart. Be sure to include all the information you will need for the bibliography page of your project.
- When you find information you can use, determine which main point the information falls under.
- Write down the information in the proper column next to the resource in which you found it.

Resources	Early Years	White House Years	Later Years
MacDonald Garrett "Who Was Grover Cleveland? <u>Historical News</u> July 29, 1985 pp. 8-16	Born Mar. 18, 1837	Democrat Served 2 terms	Died June 24 1908

TAKING NOTES
FROM WRITTEN RESOURCES

When you find a written resource that has information you can use, try following these easy steps.

1. Look in the table of contents and the index to find the sections related to your topic.
2. Read one section through. As you find useful information, mark the place with a paper clip.
3. Go through the section a second time. Think about the main points of your project.
4. If you can use the information, summarize it in your own words on your note card, topic sheet, or note chart.
5. Do this with each section of the resource.

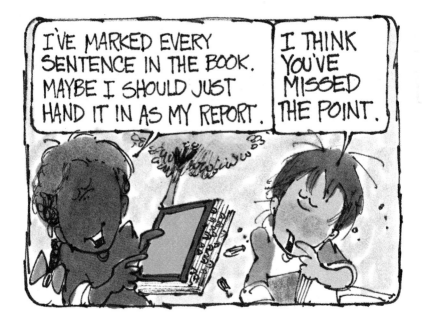

TAKING NOTES AT AN INTERVIEW

When you are using an interview as a resource,
try these suggestions:
1. Get organized ahead of time.
   - Have plenty of paper and sharpened pencils
     ready.
   - Make up a list of questions that you need
     answered.
2. Listen carefully and take careful notes.
3. Make sure all your questions are answered
   before you leave.
4. Thank the person and credit him or her in
   your report.

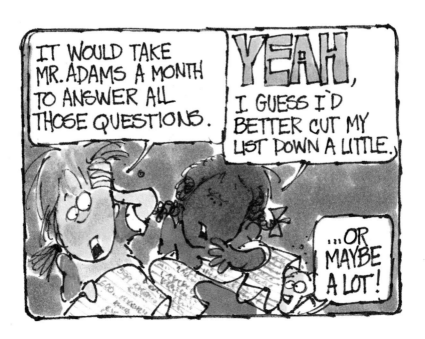

No matter which notetaking system you choose or what types of resources you use, there are some basic rules you should follow.

- Always try to write clearly.
- Study one resource at a time and go over your notes before moving on to another resource.
- Be brief. Try to limit each note to one or two sentences.
- Take notes only on information that is related to your topic.
- Copy quotes exactly including punctuation.
- Except for quotes, write down information in your own words. This lets you know that you understand the information. It also saves you from having to rewrite the information later.
- If your notes don't agree, check a third source.

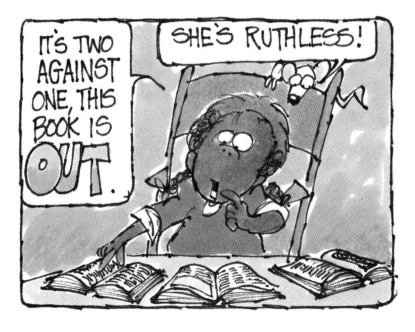

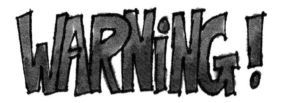

If you learn the notetaking skills in this book, your schoolwork will become easier, and...

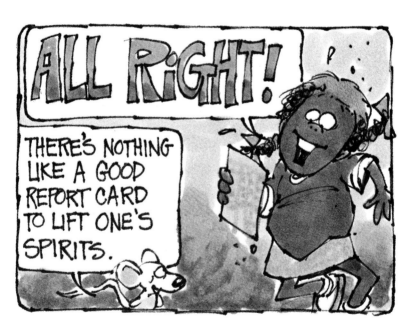

...you will probably become a better student!

THE END

About the Author

Marilyn Berry has a master's degree in education with a specialization in reading. She is on staff as a producer and creator of supplementary materials at the Institute of Living Skills. Marilyn is a published author of books and composer of music for children. She is the mother of two sons, John and Brent.